HERBAL REMEDIES FOR VARICOSE VEINS

Empower Your Veins Naturally With Herbal Medicine For Holistic Wellness, Effective Relief And Vibrant Health

DR. CARDEN KYRIE

DISCLAIMER

The only goal of this book is informational. Every effort has been taken by the author and publisher to ensure that the information provided is accurate. But the material in this book is given "as is," without any express or implied representation, warranty, or condition as to its accuracy, completeness, or suitability for any particular purpose.

Any loss, damage, or injury resulting from using the information in this book, or from any action or decision made as a result of such use, will not be covered by the author's or publisher's liability. It is recommended that readers seek the assistance of a certified specialist for guidance specific to their situation.

The opinions and viewpoints conveyed in this book belong to the author and may not necessarily represent the official stance or policies of any specified organizations or people. Any likeness to real-life occurrences, places, or people—living or deceased—is wholly coincidental.

No specific product, service, or therapy discussed in this book is endorsed by the author or publisher. Any reference to goods or services is made only for informative reasons and is not intended as a recommendation or endorsement.

Before making any judgments or acting on any information, readers are urged to independently confirm it all. Any unfavorable effects or repercussions arising from the usage of the material included in this book are disclaimed by the author and publisher.

By using this book, you consent to absolving the publisher and author of any and all claims, obligations, or losses resulting from your use of the material in it.

I appreciate your cooperation and understanding.

TABLE OF CONTENTS

CHAPTER ONE

INTRODUCTION TO VARICOSE VEINS

AN OVERVIEW OF VARICOSE VEINS

A common vascular disorder known as varicose veins refers to swollen and twisted veins that frequently have a dark purple or bluish appearance on the skin's surface. This disorder, which mostly affects the legs, is brought on by weakening or breaking vein walls and valves. The vital job of returning blood to the heart is carried out by veins; when these valves malfunction, blood accumulates in the veins, causing them to dilate and develop varicose veins. Varicose veins are more common in older adults, affecting both men and women, albeit the latter are more likely to experience them. Pregnancy, heredity, obesity, and extended standing or sitting all play a role in the development of varicose veins. Varicose veins can cause discomfort, agony, and in severe cases, consequences including ulcers or blood clots, even though they are typically thought of as a cosmetic concern.

The importance of herbal medicines has come to light in the quest to treat varicose veins and the symptoms that accompany them. Herbal remedies provide an alternative or supplementary approach to conventional medical treatments. They are produced from a variety of plants and natural components. Herbal therapies have the important benefit of being able to relieve symptoms without causing the negative side effects that are sometimes connected to pharmaceutical interventions. Herbal remedies for varicose veins frequently contain ingredients like grape seed extract, butcher's broom, and horse chestnut, which are said to improve blood flow, fortify vein walls, and lessen irritation. Herbal medicines' holistic approach fits perfectly with the public's growing interest in sustainable, natural healthcare options.

THE VALUE OF HERBAL TREATMENTS

Herbal medicines have a greater significance than just maybe curing varicose veins. Many people look to alternative therapies to manage their health, taking into account cultural influences, personal preferences, and a desire for more preventative and holistic methods. Drawing from decades of knowledge and practice, herbal medicines are frequently firmly ingrained in traditional medicine systems around the world. Their historical background makes them more appealing to people who want a safe, all-natural approach to healthcare. In addition, the growing acceptance of herbal therapies for a range of medical issues, including varicose veins, can be attributed to the desire for chemical-free solutions and environmental sustainability.

Varicose veins are a prevalent vascular disorder that has effects that go beyond aesthetics. Recognizing the physiological elements that contribute to the development of varicose veins as well as the possible consequences that may arise from this condition is essential to understanding the history of this condition. Herbal remedies are valuable in the management of varicose veins because they provide a holistic and natural alternative to conventional medical treatments. They can alleviate symptoms and may have advantages over conventional treatments, such as fewer side effects and compliance with traditional medical practices. In the complex world of treating varicose veins, herbal medicines stand out as a useful choice as people look into a variety of options for their health and well-being.

CHAPTER TWO

KNOWING ABOUT VARICOSE VEINS

MEANING AND REASONS

Legs are the most common location for varicose veins, which are swollen, twisted veins that frequently appear blue or dark purple. When the valves that control blood flow malfunction, these veins turn varicose. Though blood cannot normally flow backward through these valves, blood can pool in the veins and cause swelling and varicose veins when the valves weaken or are broken. Because standing or walking puts more strain on the lower extremities, this ailment most often affects the legs.

Varicose veins can occur due to several circumstances. Age is a major factor, as veins become less elastic with age and are more likely to expand. In addition, genetic predisposition contributes, with a family history of varicose veins raising the risk of the ailment.

Another reason is gender, since women are more prone to varicose veins, particularly during menopause and other hormonal changes. Varicose veins can also develop as a result of obesity, long stretches of standing or sitting, and a sedentary lifestyle.

HAZARD CONTRIBUTORS

Varicose veins are more likely to form if certain risk factors are met. A family history of the illness is one example of a hereditary component that might greatly increase the risk. Another significant risk factor is gender; women are more likely to develop varicose veins than men, in part because of hormonal changes that occur during menstruation, pregnancy, and menopause. Age is a factor, and as people age, their risk increases.

The risk is increased by obesity and inactivity, which both increase the strain on veins. Varicose veins can also be more common in occupations that require extended standing or sitting, such as those in the medical field or the workplace.

INDICATIONS AND ADVERSE EVENTS

Varicose veins usually cause moderate symptoms at first, but as they worsen, they can cause more serious issues. Leg pain that aches or throbs, a feeling of weight or discomfort, and visible, twisted veins immediately beneath the skin are common symptoms. Another typical symptom is swelling, especially after extended periods of sitting or standing. Untreated varicose veins may result in complications.

One possible consequence is chronic venous insufficiency, which is defined as the veins' incapacity to return enough blood to the heart. In more advanced cases, skin abnormalities including pigmentation or the emergence of ulcers may happen. Furthermore, varicose veins may develop superficial thrombophlebitis, a disorder involving the production of blood clots, which presents additional health problems.

Varicose veins are a common vascular disorder that typically affects the legs and is characterized by swollen, twisted veins. Their development is influenced by several variables, such as age, gender, heredity, and lifestyle decisions. It is essential to comprehend the risk factors to prevent and take early action. It's critical to identify varicose vein symptoms, such as pain, swelling, and visible veins, because if left untreated, they can result in consequences including superficial thrombophlebitis and chronic venous insufficiency. By modifying one's lifestyle and seeking medical counsel, varicose vein symptoms can be managed and lessened, improving vascular health in general.

CHAPTER THREE

TRADITIONAL INTERVENTIONS
MEDICAL OPERATIONS

Medical procedures, which include a broad range of treatments aimed at diagnosing, treating, or preventing various medical problems, are essential to the healthcare industry. To improve or restore a person's health, these treatments frequently entail the use of specialist methods, tools, and technologies. Treatment of vascular problems, such as varicose veins, is one prominent area where medical techniques are often used.

SCLEROTHERAPY

A minimally invasive medical method used to treat spider and varicose veins is called sclerotherapy. A specific fluid, usually a saline solution or a chemical irritant, is injected directly into the veins that are damaged during this operation. By causing the veins to collapse and eventually disappear, the injected solution reroutes blood flow to healthier veins. Smaller veins near the skin's surface respond best to sclerosing therapy. For people looking to address the esthetic and discomfort aspects of varicose veins, it is a commonly used and generally well-tolerated treatment option.

LASER TREATMENT

Another medical procedure used to treat varicose veins is laser therapy, sometimes referred to as endovenous laser treatment (EVLT) or endovenous laser ablation. With this method, the damaged veins are heated and sealed shut using laser radiation. A little tube is used to inject a laser fiber into the vein that is giving you trouble throughout the treatment. The laser produces heat when it is turned on, which closes the vein. Blood is redirected through healthier veins as the body eventually absorbs the blocked vein. Because it leaves fewer scars and requires less time to recover from than traditional surgical methods, laser therapy is frequently regarded as a less invasive option.

STRIPPING THE VEINS

A more conventional surgical method for treating varicose veins is vein stripping, which is usually saved for more serious situations. A surgeon creates skin incisions and extracts, or "strips," the damaged vein from the leg during this treatment. Vein stripping has been around for a while, but its use has decreased as less invasive methods like sclerotherapy and laser therapy have advanced. These more recent techniques frequently offer equivalent effectiveness with less invasiveness, resulting in quicker recovery periods and fewer side effects.

There are several ways to treat varicose veins, including sclerotherapy, laser therapy, and vein stripping. The degree of the ailment, the patient's preferences, and the advice of medical experts all influence the method that is chosen. These interventions highlight how medical procedures are always evolving, with a focus on less invasive methods to improve patient results and happiness.

CHAPTER FOUR

MODIFICATIONS IN LIFESTYLE

EXERCISE

A healthy lifestyle is based on regular physical activity, which has many advantages beyond improved physical fitness. Exercise is essential for preserving ideal cardiovascular health, controlling weight, and improving general well-being. A well-rounded fitness regimen incorporates a variety of exercises, such as strength training, flexibility training, and cardiovascular sports like swimming or running.

Exercise is important for lowering the risk of chronic illnesses including heart disease, diabetes, and some types of cancer in addition to helping people maintain a healthy weight.

In addition, regular exercise improves mental health by reducing stress, anxiety, and sadness. Physical activity causes endorphins to be released, which enhances happiness and well-being.

Exercise doesn't have to be strenuous to be a part of daily life; modest exercises like cycling or brisk walking can have a big impact on one's general health. The secret is to identify sustainable and pleasurable activities that will encourage a long-term commitment to an active lifestyle.

COMPRESSION STOCKINGS

Compression stockings are becoming more and more well-known for their therapeutic uses, especially in promoting better circulation and averting a range of vascular problems. The upward circulation of blood into the heart is facilitated by the moderate pressure these specifically made stockings impart to the legs. By keeping blood from accumulating in the veins, this compression lowers the chance of developing diseases including venous insufficiency and deep vein thrombosis (DVT). Compression stockings are frequently advised for people with certain medical concerns, such as varicose veins, as well as those who spend a lot of time sitting or standing.

Compression stockings have more and more uses outside of medicine in the sports and fitness industries. Compression stockings can help athletes—particularly those in endurance sports—reduce discomfort in their muscles, increase blood flow, and speed up recovery from strenuous exercise. Even though wearing compression stockings is typically safe, it's important to speak with a healthcare provider to figure out the right amount and level of compression for your particular needs.

DIETARY ADVICE

The foundation of general health and well-being is a well-rounded, nutrient-dense diet. Dietary decisions are vital for maintaining good body functions and preventing chronic diseases in addition to having an impact on weight management. Meeting nutritional demands requires a focus on a range of nutrient-dense foods, such as fruits, vegetables, whole grains, lean meats, and healthy fats. For instance, the Mediterranean diet, which emphasizes a high intake of vegetables, seafood, and olive oil, is well known for its health advantages.

A better relationship with food is also facilitated by mindful eating techniques like savoring every meal and paying attention to portion sizes. Preventing obesity, diabetes, and cardiovascular diseases requires limiting the use of processed foods, sugar-filled drinks, and high amounts of saturated and trans fats. Another essential component of a healthy diet is being properly hydrated, since water aids in digestion, nutrition absorption, and general body functions.

Dietary modifications can be more long-term sustainable if they are made gradually as opposed to drastically. Speaking with a licensed dietitian may provide a well-rounded and nourishing approach to food by offering individualized advice based on each person's nutritional needs and health objectives.

CHAPTER FIVE

OVERVIEW OF HERBAL REMEDIES

TRADITIONALLY, HERBS WERE USED FOR HEALING

Herbs have been used historically by humans to promote and preserve health. Herbs have been used medicinally from the dawn of time when different societies gained a profound awareness of the healing qualities of plants. For instance, the Shen Nong Ben Cao Jing and other ancient Chinese writings describe the applications of hundreds of herbs, making traditional herbal medicine a fundamental component of treatment techniques in that region. In a similar vein, records indicate that the ancient Egyptians used plants like garlic and aloe vera to treat a variety of illnesses.

Herbalism was very popular in medieval Europe when monks kept large herb gardens for therapeutic purposes. Herbal knowledge was frequently passed down through families or communities over several generations.

With a strong affinity for plants, Native American cultures used echinacea and goldenseal for their therapeutic benefits. The varied ways that various cultures have used nature's healing powers are reflected in the complex tapestry of historical herbal use.

SAFETY & SAFETY MEASURES

Herbal treatments provide a natural approach to health and well-being, but it's important to recognize that there may be hazards involved. Herbal treatments' safety is dependent on several factors, such as the particular herb used, how it is prepared, and the patient's health status. One should not ignore factors like drug interactions, allergic responses, and the possibility of toxicity.

Herbal treatments are safe to use, but before adding them into a wellness program, especially if one is pregnant, nursing, or on prescription medicine, one should speak with a certified healthcare expert.

Because some herbs may have adverse effects or contraindications, it's critical to use them responsibly and with knowledge. To prevent negative effects, appropriate dosage and preparation are also essential.

HOW HERBAL MEDICINES FUNCTION

The intricate chemical components found in plants are responsible for the medicinal effectiveness of herbal treatments. These substances, which include essential oils, flavonoids, and alkaloids, provide herbs with their therapeutic qualities. These bioactive substances interact with the human body in different ways, which result in different physiological reactions.

Herbs can affect the body's immune, circulatory, and neurological systems, among other systems. Herbs such as valerian root may have a relaxing impact on the nervous system, while echinacea is thought to stimulate the immune system. Numerous herbal medicines have antibacterial, anti-inflammatory, and antioxidant qualities that help them treat a variety of medical conditions.

Herbal medicine's holistic approach recognizes the body's connection to the environment. Herbal treatments frequently complement the body's natural processes synergistically, aiding in the restoration of harmony and balance. The mechanisms of action behind herbal treatments are still being investigated by science, which helps to clarify their possible advantages and deepens our knowledge of how these age-old healing methods relate to contemporary medical techniques.

CHAPTER SIX

HERBS FOR SWOLLEN LEGS

THE AESCULUS HIPPOCASTANUM, OR HORSE CHESTNUT

The popular herb horse chestnut, scientifically known as Aesculus hippocastanum, has long been used to treat varicose veins and associated circulation problems. Aescin, a substance found in horse chestnut tree seeds, is thought to have anti-inflammatory and vein-strengthening qualities.

Benefits and Uses: Improving blood circulation and reducing leg swelling, a typical indication of varicose veins, are two of horse chestnut's main advantages. It is believed that asecin increases blood vessel flexibility, which enhances vein function. Furthermore, this herb is frequently used to relieve varicose vein symptoms like discomfort and heaviness.

Administration and Dosage: Horse chestnut extract is advised to be taken at different times of day, but typically between 300 and 600 mg. Since every person's needs are unique, it is imperative to speak with a healthcare provider before beginning any supplementation. To guarantee constant potency, the extract is usually standardized to include a given proportion of aescin.

RUMEX ACULEATUS, OFTEN KNOWN AS BUTCHER'S BROOM

Ruscus aculeatus, scientifically known as Butcher's Broom, is another herbal treatment that has been used historically to treat circulation problems, such as varicose veins. Active ingredients found in this evergreen plant include ruscogenins, which are thought to have anti-inflammatory and vasoconstrictive properties.

Uses and Benefits: Butcher's broom is well known for its ability to strengthen blood vessels and lower inflammation, especially when venous insufficiency is present. It is frequently used to treat varicose vein symptoms like leg cramps, edema, and itching. Better blood flow and less vein pooling may be attributed to the vasoconstrictive qualities.

Administration and Dosage: Although there are no set guidelines for the dosage of Butcher's Broom, a typical range is between 100 and 300 mg of the standardized extract per day. Following a doctor's advice is essential while using any herbal product, as it can provide insight into specific medical concerns and possible drug interactions.

CENTELLA ASIATICA, OR GOTU KOLA

Centella Asiatica, also known as gotu kola, is a herb with a long history of use in traditional medicine. It is said to offer several health advantages, including support for circulatory health.

Uses and Benefits: Gotu Kola is known to strengthen connective tissues and increase the formation of collagen, both of which may improve vein flexibility. This herb is frequently used to reduce swelling and irritation that are related to varicose veins. It is also believed to promote general vascular health.

Dosage & Administration: Although there are no set guidelines for Gotu Kola extract dosage, a typical range is between 60 and 120 mg daily. It is essential to speak with a healthcare professional to figure out the right dosage depending on a person's specific medical needs and any possible contraindications.

KNOWN AS HAMAMELIS VIRGINIANA, WITCH HAZEL

Scientifically called Hamamelis virginiana, witch hazel is a multipurpose herb with astringent qualities that have been used historically to treat a variety of skin and circulation conditions.

Benefits and Applications: Witch Hazel is prized for its capacity to tone blood vessels and lessen inflammation. By narrowing blood vessels and decreasing edema, it is thought to relieve pain brought on by varicose veins when given topically. For a synergistic effect, it can also be used in combination with other herbs.

Dosage and Administration: Ointments or distilled liquids containing witch hazel are frequently administered topically. It is frequently applied externally to the afflicted areas as an herbal treatment for varicose veins. Nonetheless, it's crucial to adhere to the directions on the product and seek the opinion of a medical expert for specialized guidance.

EXTRACT FROM PINE BARK (PINUS PINASTER)

The maritime pine tree (Pinus pinaster) is the source of pine bark extract, which is known for its strong antioxidant qualities and has drawn interest due to its possible advantages in treating circulatory problems.

Advantages and Applications: Proanthocyanidins, one of the active ingredients in pine bark extract, are thought to strengthen blood vessels and enhance circulation in general.

This makes it a viable choice for those with varicose veins because it might help lessen uncomfortable and swollen sensations. Furthermore, its antioxidant qualities might aid in preventing oxidative stress on blood vessels.

Dosage and Administration: Between 100 and 300 mg per day is the usual range of dosage recommendations for pine bark extract. Selecting a standardized extract is crucial to guarantee constant concentrations of active ingredients. As with other herbal supplements, it is best to speak with a healthcare provider to ascertain the right dosage depending on personal health concerns and any drug interactions.

CHAPTER SEVEN

HERBAL FORMULAS AND COMBINATIONS

SYNERGISTIC IMPACT OF HERBS

Herbal combinations have synergistic effects that are vital to both conventional and complementary medicine methods. The idea that the combination action of various herbs can boost therapeutic advantages beyond what each herb can achieve individually is one that herbalists frequently emphasize. This synergy results from the intricate interactions between the many active components in the herbs, which have a more balanced and comprehensive effect on the body. Certain herb combos can reduce adverse effects, while other combinations may improve the effectiveness or absorption of one herb. Herbalists can formulate remedies that target certain health issues because of their understanding of the synergistic effects, which necessitates a thorough understanding of the characteristics and actions of various plants.

COMBINATIONS OF HERBS FOR VARICOSE VEINS

A common health problem is varicose veins, which are characterized by twisted, enlarged veins, generally in the legs. The main goals of herbal remedies for varicose veins are frequently to increase blood vessel wall strength, lower irritation, and improve circulation. Because horse chestnut (Aesculus hippocastanum) is well-known for promoting venous health, it is often added to these formulations. Horse chestnut's bioactive ingredients, such as aescin, aid in toning veins and lessen edema. Herbs known to improve blood flow and decrease inflammation in the affected areas, such as butcher's broom (Ruscus aculeatus) and gotu kola (Centella Asiatica), are also frequently included.

FORMULA EXAMPLES

A mixture of butcher's broom, gotu kola, and horse chestnut is one example of an herbal remedy for varicose veins. By utilizing the synergistic benefits of these herbs, this blend offers complete support for the health of your arteries. Not only does horse chestnut have anti-inflammatory and vein-strengthening qualities, but butcher's broom and gotu kola enhance microcirculation and minimize swelling. There are other ways to make the formulation, including tincture, pill, or tea, so people can select a method that fits their needs and schedule.

HOW TO PREPARE AND USE IT

The qualities of each herb and the intended medicinal results are carefully taken into account while creating herbal formulations and combinations. To produce a tincture for varicose veins, one could macerate dry plants in alcohol to extract their active ingredients. Alternatively, the dry herbs can be steeped to make a tea or decoction. To guarantee safety and effectiveness when preparing herbs, it is imperative to adhere to established rules. When using herbal remedies for varicose veins, there are usually guidelines regarding dosage, frequency, and length of use.

It is recommended to regularly monitor the results and seek advice from a licensed herbalist or healthcare provider to evaluate the effectiveness of the herbal regimen and make any required modifications. Including these measures in a complete strategy that may also involve lifestyle changes will help to improve the overall effectiveness and management of varicose veins.

CHAPTER EIGHT

USING HERBAL REMEDIES IN EVERYDAY SITUATIONS

HERBAL INFUSIONS AND TEAS

A pleasant approach to get the benefits of the medicinal characteristics of many plants is to incorporate herbal teas and infusions into your daily routine. Herbal teas come in a variety of flavors and have healing properties. They are made from dried leaves, flowers, seeds, or roots. For instance, chamomile tea is well known for its relaxing qualities, which make it a great option for reducing stress and encouraging deeper sleep. Conversely, peppermint tea is renowned for its flavor and digestive properties. People can customize their choices according to their health needs and personal preferences by experimenting with various herbal mixtures.

Herbal infusions are prepared by steeping herbs in hot water, which releases their therapeutic properties. This process guarantees that the medicinal qualities of the herbs are successfully infused into the drink while also enhancing their flavor. Herbal teas are an easy yet effective method to focus holistic well-being in your daily routine, whether it's a morning ritual or an evening wind-down.

TOPICAL APPLICATIONS

Herbal treatments can be applied topically to incorporate them into daily life, in addition to their ingestion. The body's largest organ, the skin, may absorb healthy chemicals from a variety of herbs. Herbal oils, balms, and salves provide a healthy substitute for store-bought skincare products. Calendula-infused oil, for example, has anti-inflammatory and skin-soothing qualities that make it a great option for soothing and hydrating sensitive skin. Aloe vera, which is frequently applied externally for its restorative and cooling properties, can be grown at home or bought as a gel to soothe sunburns.

Herbs may offer an additional layer of regeneration and relaxation to both practices. Relaxing baths with Epsom salt infused with lavender or chamomile can help reduce stress and promote muscular relaxation. During such techniques, the herbal ingredients are absorbed through the skin, supporting a holistic approach to health and well-being.

NUTRITIONAL GUIDELINES

Herbal medicines can be incorporated into daily life in a way that emphasizes a balanced and comprehensive approach, including food choices. Herbs used in cooking, such as basil, rosemary, and thyme, have additional health advantages in addition to improving food flavor. Antioxidants and other micronutrients that support general health are abundant in these herbs. For instance, the Mediterranean diet emphasizes the use of herbs in cooking, associating tasty food with healthful qualities.

Herbal supplements can also be incorporated into a regular diet to help with specific health issues or nutritional deficiencies. Due to their well-known anti-inflammatory qualities, supplements containing turmeric are frequently used to promote joint health. People can design a complete and customized approach to nutrition that supports their health objectives by combining nutrient-dense diets with herbal supplements.

HERBAL LIFESTYLE RECOMMENDATIONS

Including herbal medicines in daily life goes beyond using certain products and involves adopting a holistic herbal way of living. This includes mindfulness exercises like herbal meditation, in which participants interact with the energies and scents of herbs to promote calmness and mental clarity. Herbalists frequently recommend spending time in the outdoors and developing a closer relationship with plants to promote harmony and balance.

Herbal gardening also turns into a healing and uplifting activity that enables people to grow their herbs for flavor, medicine, or decoration

CHAPTER NINE

WAY OF LIFE AND PREVENTIVE STEPS

EXERCISE AND PHYSICAL ACTIVITY

These activities are essential for maintaining general health and preventing several diseases. Numerous health benefits, such as better cardiovascular health, improved mood, and more energy, have been linked to physical activity. Adults should strive to engage in muscle-strengthening exercises two or more days a week in addition to 150 minutes of moderate-intensity aerobic activity or 75 minutes of vigorous-intensity aerobic activity per week. Numerous exercises, such as brisk walking, jogging, cycling, or playing sports, can help achieve this.

SUSTAINING A HEALTHY WEIGHT

Remaining at a healthy weight is essential for avoiding heart disease, diabetes, and some types of cancer, among other illnesses. Health and weight control have a complicated relationship that depends on several variables, including genetics, physical activity, and food. Having a healthy, well-balanced diet and exercising frequently help with weight control.

It's critical to place equal emphasis on developing healthful habits that promote overall well-being as well as the number on the scale. Seeking advice from dietitians or medical specialists might offer tailored recommendations for reaching and sustaining a healthy weight.

HANDLING STRESS

Although stress is an inevitable aspect of life, prolonged stress can be harmful to one's physical and emotional well-being. The detrimental effects of chronic stress must be avoided by putting into practice efficient stress management strategies. Techniques like yoga, deep breathing exercises, mindfulness meditation, and getting enough sleep can all help reduce stress and foster serenity. Developing solid social ties and preserving a good work-life balance are also crucial aspects of stress management. Early identification and resolution of stressors can have a substantial positive impact on long-term well-being.

STEER CLEAR OF EXTENDED STANDING OR SITTING

Prolonged sitting or standing can exacerbate several health concerns, such as cardiovascular and musculoskeletal disorders, as we lead increasingly sedentary lifestyles. It is advised to include mobility into everyday routines and to intersperse brief periods of standing or sitting with longer ones. Prolonged static positions can be less harmful if simple movements like stretching, walking, or mild exercise are done regularly. To reduce the possibility of discomfort and support musculoskeletal health, ergonomic factors must be taken into account in both sitting and standing work situations. Maintaining a healthy balance between sitting, standing, and moving throughout the day is essential to avoiding the negative consequences linked to extended periods of inactivity.

CHAPTER TEN

SPEAKING WITH MEDICAL EXPERTS

WHEN TO GET EXPERT COUNSEL

It is imperative to consult a specialist for assistance regarding matters of health and well-being. Maintaining good health and taking care of possible medical issues requires knowing when to seek advice from medical professionals. Persistent or increasing symptoms are one of the main signs that you should consult a doctor. It becomes essential to see a healthcare provider if someone has symptoms that do not get better or get worse over time.

Preventive care and regular examinations are also essential components of healthcare. Even in the absence of symptoms, routine medical checkups help in the early identification and treatment of possible health problems. Preventive measures and timely intervention are essential elements in preserving general health. People should prioritize preventive healthcare to stop the development of more dangerous conditions rather than waiting until they are quite ill to see medical specialists.

Getting professional assistance in the context of pre-existing medical issues is another crucial factor to take into account. People who have continuing medical issues or chronic illnesses should stay in regular contact with their healthcare professionals. This makes it possible to rapidly address any changes in symptoms or treatment plans, thereby maximizing the care of the underlying ailment.

COMBINING MEDICAL TREATMENTS WITH HERBAL REMEDIES

The question of combining herbal medicines with medical treatments needs to be carefully considered and discussed with medical authorities. Although the potential health advantages of herbal remedies have been used for generations in many cultures, caution must be exercised when integrating them with medical therapy.

A person's health may be significantly impacted by the combination of conventional drugs and herbs.

When it comes to educating patients about the safe and efficient use of herbal remedies in addition to medical therapies, healthcare professionals are essential. They can shed light on possible interactions between herbs and drugs, preventing side effects or compromising the effectiveness of prescription drugs. Furthermore, healthcare providers can assist people in navigating the wide range of herbal products on the market and point them in the direction of reliable and evidence-based choices.

Open communication between patients and healthcare providers is also necessary for the integration of herbal therapies with medical treatments. People should disclose to their medical providers all information regarding any herbal supplements they use, including the quantity and frequency of use. Using the full picture of a patient's health, healthcare providers can make well-informed decisions on treatment plans with the use of this information.

Consulting a professional is essential to preserving and improving one's health. Consulting with healthcare professionals guarantees a holistic approach to well-being, whether it means treating chronic diseases, addressing persistent symptoms, or giving preventive care priority. Working together with healthcare experts becomes even more important when contemplating the combination of herbal remedies with medical therapies. A balanced and individualized approach to healthcare is enhanced by open communication and well-informed decision-making, which improves outcomes for those looking to integrate herbal therapies into a comprehensive wellness plan.